contents

T0201034

The role of the mentor is multifaceted and can be demanding. This guidance aims to offer the mentor practical advice on how to meet the challenges they may face in order to fulfil this exciting and dynamic role. Mentorship has a unique place in preparing the next generation of professionals and as such the mentor role is key to the teaching, learning and assessment processes within the practice setting.

The rationale for producing this pocket book is to produce a readily available guide for mentors who are supporting students in a work placement. Many mentors will have undertaken preparation prior to commencing their role whilst others will have entered into the role by nature of their professional work experience. This guide will examine the key areas within the role and offer practical advice on how to establish and maintain quality placements which provide an optimum learning environment for students in healthcare. It is envisaged that the points raised will stimulate further reading.

Many professions operate some form of mentorship within their workplace environment and it is recognised that there are specific standards and guidance related to the mentor role such as the College of Operating Department Practitioners (CODP) (2009) document. This guide is based upon the standards published by the Nursing & Midwifery Council (NMC) (2008). This is to offer structure to the guide and should not act as a barrier to mentors from other professions utilising the guide. It is the intention of the authors that the guide will offer support to mentors from any profession. The issues examined in the guide are generic and applicable to mentors from all professional fields. It is acknowledged that each profession will utilise its own terms for supervisors of students. Due to the inter-professional focus throughout the guide, the terms 'student' and 'mentor' will be adopted in order to present a generic approach.

References / College of Operating Department Practitioners (2009) *Standards, recommendations and guidance for mentors and practice placements.* London: CODP; Nursing & Midwifery Council (2008) *Standards to support learning and assessment in practice.* London: NMC.

Planning for your student

Good mentors need leadership and planning skills to enhance student learning. Therefore, before they arrive in the placement it is important to find out the student's name, level of study and when they will be arriving. This will help you develop a learning experience which meets the needs of the student and enhances the learning experience. The aim is to ensure students will feel welcome and ready to learn.

When planning for the student to arrive a mentor should:
- Contact the student with information on where and what time to arrive.
- Provide the student with the name of the mentor who will undertake the supervision.
- Provide written information about the work/placement area.

■ FIRST DAY

The mentor should:
- Plan to be available to greet the student.
- Introduce the student to the team.
- Orientate the student to the work area, including policies, procedure and health and safety issues, e.g. fire regulations.
- Discuss the required aims and learning outcomes for the placement.

■ A KEY FUNCTION OF A MENTOR IS TO BE AN EFFECTIVE LEADER

A good leader should:
- Plan a series of learning experiences to enable the student to meet the required learning outcomes.
- Act as an advocate to facilitate learning.
- Act as a role model.
- Prioritise work in order to allow time to support students.
- Delegate tasks in accordance with the student's level of study.

Reference / Gopee, N. (2008) *Mentoring and supervision in healthcare*. London: Sage Publications.

Establishing a relationship

The student–mentor relationship invariably draws on emotion. Mentors want their students to be successful and may feel personally responsible if they fail. Students often see their mentors as a 'nurturing' or 'parental' figure, which may put additional pressure on the mentor. While it is important to recognise the personal aspects of the relationship as a mentor you must remember that you have multiple roles, which can be conflicting particularly if summative assessment is part of your mentoring role (Wilkes 2006).

Reference / Wilkes, Z. (2006) The student–mentor relationship: a review of the literature. *Nursing Standard* **20** (37), 42–7.

Developing an effective professional relationship will provide valuable experiential learning for students and a stimulating, rewarding career for you as a mentor.

■ COMMUNICATION

Communication is the key to any relationship and it is essential to establish a two-way communication system from the beginning.

A good mentor should:
1. Communicate in a style which aids clear understanding.
2. Avoid using jargon and specific terminology that is not easily understood.
3. Be aware of appropriate non-verbal communication, i.e. body language and eye contact.

4. Use open questions to elicit more in-depth communication.
5. Allow the student time to express their thoughts and feelings and listen to their concerns.
6. Be clear about what you want to say and be unambiguous.
7. Always consider the environment where the communication is taking place, e.g. you may need to find a quiet environment where you cannot be overheard.

■ GROUND RULES

Setting ground rules for the duration of the placement helps to establish exactly what is expected of everyone involved and could be developed into a learning contract.

Ground rules could include issues such as:
- Arriving on time.
- Listening to others.
- Acknowledging when you do not understand.
- Treating others with respect.
- Maintaining confidentiality.
- Establishing time for reflection and asking questions.

Reference / http://www.faculty.londondeanery.ac.uk/e-learning/small-group-teaching/setting-ground-rules

■ OBJECTIVITY IN A RELATIONSHIP

('It's not you, it's me')

Inevitably you will establish a relationship with your student: as with any relationship it can be emotive, but mentors must be fair and treat all students with equity. It is therefore important to ensure that your relationship with your student enables you to be objective. You will inevitably meet students you get attached to and of course you will meet others whom you do not get on with easily. It is important to take this into account so that you avoid individual bias. This is known as the Halo/Horn effect and refers to a tendency to give a student higher or lower marks because of the impression they have made on you (Walsh 2010).

Reference / Walsh, D. (2010) *The nurse mentor's handbook: supporting students in clinical practice.* Berkshire: Open University Press.

■ *THINK!*

Consider the following factors:

- **Compatibility**
  Halo – we find pleasing people who agree with us and we evaluate them more highly.
- **The high potential effect**
  Halo – we often judge a person's credentials rather than what they have actually done, hence the person with the good looks or advanced degrees rates higher.
- **The 'no complaint' bias**
  Halo – a tendency to treat no news as good, so if there have been no complaints it is assumed that everything is fine.
- **The contrary person**
  Horn – we can become irritated with people who disagree with us on too many things and reflect this in our judgement of them.

- **The effect of a person's past record**
  Halo and horn – we sometimes assume that because a person has done some good work in the past, everything is satisfactory, or alternatively we assume that if there have been problems, these will continue.
- **Central tendency**
  Halo and horn – sometimes the assessor worries about the consequences of giving high or low marks and avoids risk by assessing everyone as average.

HINTS
- Develop a very clear understanding of the nature of each learning outcome and the kind of behaviour it describes. You will then have a clear idea of what you expect of the student.
- Pay attention to the student's all-round performance. When an individual is particularly impressive or disappointing in one area avoid the tendency to categorise all other performance the same.
- Focus on the differences, not similarities, between you. What transferable skills and qualities does the student bring with them?
- Gather as much information as you can, and do not let a single experience determine your opinion of a student's performance.
- Maintain your own portfolio/records and reflect on your input to the student's achievement.

■ LEARNING STYLES

Everyone has their own preferred approach to learning. For example some students may prefer to learn by watching a procedure and then undertaking it themselves. Alternatively they may prefer to read about the process before they undertake it. To enhance the learning experience a mentor needs to discuss or assess how the student prefers to learn.

You should discuss the student's preferred method and style of learning to facilitate the learning process.

A mentor should identify what type of learner their student is:

- Activist: learns by becoming involved and doing.
- Pragmatist: learns by tackling problems.
- Theorist: learns by reading and reviewing.
- Reflector: learns by thinking and watching.

Reference / Honey, P. and Mumford, A. (2000) *The Learning Style Helper's Guide.* Maidenhead: Peter Honey.

What type of learner are you?

When you buy a new piece of technology, for instance a mobile telephone, do you

a) Read the instructions before you try to use the phone.

b) Learn how to operate the phone by using it.

If you answered (a) you are likely to be a theorist (or reflector) as you like to read about or think about something before you engage in the activity.

If you answered (b) you are likely to be an activist (or pragmatist) as you like to get involved and use actions to solve a problem.

Teaching strategies

When you have identified your own learning style and that of your student you then need to consider what teaching style you will adopt to meet your student's learning needs. Basically there are two fundamental approaches to teaching. One is **pedagogy** where the mentor takes charge and leads the student through the learning process. Here the student will be dependent upon the approaches, attitudes and actions of the mentor. The mentor will decide what the student learns and how. This may be appropriate in some situations, for example when there is only one way to carry out a task or procedure, such as in an emergency situation. The other approach is **andragogy** as identified by Knowles (1994) where the student is put at the centre of the learning process. Here the mentor will see each student as an individual. The mentor will then facilitate learning opportunities which will enable each student to achieve to their potential. The mentor needs to guide a student's learning but this is based upon the student's past experiences and knowledge level. The mentor will negotiate learning opportunities with the student. This approach will help develop students who can problem solve and engage in self-regulated learning.

Reference / Knowles, M. (1994) *The Adult Learner: a neglected species*, 4th edn. Houston: Gulf Publications.

■ LEARNING THEORIES

As Bloom (1956) states, all learning brings about a change in behaviour and this takes place in three domains:
- Cognitive – intellectual ability and knowledge.
- Psychomotor – skills and performance.
- Affective – behaviour and attitude.

Think about learning to drive as an example.

A learner driver is taught how to accelerate, change the gears, brake, indicate, steer and reverse but performing these skills (**psychomotor domain**) is not enough. They should also understand why they have to change gear or indicate and learn the rules or laws which apply to using the road (**cognitive domain**). Furthermore they must also behave appropriately so that they do not impede other road users and are able to judge situations effectively, valuing fellow drivers (**affective domain**).

As a mentor therefore you must ensure that your student has developed their learning in each of the domains and plan your teaching strategies accordingly. Learning theories are the tools you can use to help you achieve this but the learning theory you use will depend upon the learning outcome you want to achieve.

Behaviourist theory

This draws on the work of Pavlov (classical conditioning) and Skinner (operant conditioning), (Snowman, McCown and Bielher 2009). Remember Pavlov's dogs and how he observed that they salivated when they were fed. He rang a bell at feeding time and eventually the dogs associated the ringing bell with food, to the point where they only had to hear the bell to salivate. Pavlov had conditioned the dogs to respond to his stimulus.

Skinner developed these ideas and argued that behaviours are reinforced when they are rewarded. He demonstrated this by rewarding a hungry rat with food when it pressed a lever. This was accidental at first but the rat soon learnt that pressing the lever brought food. Skinner developed the experiment so that the food only appeared at times when specific conditions supported pressing the lever, for example, when a low frequency was heard. The rat therefore was conditioned to operate the lever and did not press the lever randomly.

Advantages – It is a successful teaching strategy as the desired behaviour is reinforced with rewards and repetition or practice ensuring that the student develops good skills. This is useful for outcomes which require the student to be able to recall information quickly or take immediate action.

Disadvantages – It does not address comprehension or understanding of the process, it becomes a reaction. The student is a passive recipient.

Social learning theory

Albert Bandura is widely recognised as the person whose work developed this approach and, like Skinner, he believed that behaviour could be reinforced but linked it to observation and imitation of a role model. His experiments demonstrated that children who observed aggressive behaviour were more likely to behave in a similar way, imitating what they had seen.

Advantages – Again as a teaching strategy it is effective as the student seeks to be as good as or better than their mentor. Motivation is high so the student learns quickly, particularly if they admire the role model and adopting the behaviour leads to a desired outcome.

Disadvantages – Self-regulation is an important component of social learning theory, otherwise students will simply copy behaviour whether it is appropriate or not.

Cognitive theory

Cognitive theorists try to determine how people learn. They explore how people think, memorise knowledge or recall events and apply that knowledge to solve problems.

Bruner suggests that the student constructs ideas or concepts by drawing on their past and new knowledge in order to make decisions. It is important therefore for the student to experience the process so that when they are involved in a similar situation they will draw on their experiences (old knowledge), assess the present situation (new knowledge), and make decisions based on their analysis of all the information that they have. Piaget's work also plays an important role in developing this theory as it utilises the principles of assimilation, accommodation and schema formation.

Advantages – It enables the student to develop the skills and qualities demanded in healthcare as that knowledge is transferable; they are able to critically analyse and problem solve.

Disadvantages – Success depends upon the amount of effort a student puts into the work and their belief in their own ability to achieve.

Humanism

The focus of the humanist is on the student to determine their own learning needs. Rogers (1969) states that all human beings have a natural potential to learn and that the teacher is a facilitator who can create the appropriate conditions for learning to occur.

Maslow (1987) established a Hierarchy of Need. He states that all the needs must be met in particular order before an individual can achieve their potential (self-actualisation).

Advantages – It makes learning meaningful to the student and can be inspirational. Students develop the skills they need to teach themselves.

Disadvantages – Mentors often feel that they have lost control of the student's learning and therefore cannot predict the learning outcomes.

References / Bloom, B.S. (1956) *Taxonomy of Education Objectives*. London: Longman; Maslow, A.H. (1987) *Motivation and Personality*, 3rd edn. New York: Harper & Row; Rogers, C.R. (1969) *Freedom to learn*. Columbus, OH: Charles E. Merrill Publishing Co.; Snowman, J., McCown, R. and Biehler, R. (2009) *Psychology applied to teaching*. Boston, MA: Houghton Mifflin.

■ INTER-PROFESSIONAL LEARNING (IPL)

Inter-professional learning takes place 'when students from two or more professions learn about, from and with each other to enable effective collaboration and improve health outcomes' (WHO 2010 p. 7).

Inter-professional learning is also known as inter-professional education and is gaining increasing recognition around the world as a way to strengthen the healthcare workforce for future generations. It develops practitioners who work together for the benefit of the patient or client, removing duplication and wasteful competition. They share best practice and support each other as health issues become increasingly challenging and complex.

Most curricula will demand that students gain a wider experience which includes time spent with other agencies and/or professions but even if it is not a mandatory learning outcome it is still best practice to offer such opportunities to your student.

■ *THINK!*

Consider the following list. How often do you contact other agencies or professions to discuss patients or clients?

Contact with other professionals

PROFESSION	FREQUENCY OF CONTACT: DAILY/ WEEKLY/ MONTHLY	CONSIDER IF YOUR STUDENTS' LEARNING CAN BE ENHANCED FROM A VISIT TO THESE DEPARTMENTS OR COULD YOU EXCHANGE STUDENTS WITH OTHER MENTORS?
Nurses		
Midwives		
Doctors		
Dieticians		
Occupational therapists		
Pharmacists		

PROFESSION	FREQUENCY OF CONTACT: DAILY/ WEEKLY/ MONTHLY	CONSIDER IF YOUR STUDENTS' LEARNING CAN BE ENHANCED FROM A VISIT TO THESE DEPARTMENTS OR COULD YOU EXCHANGE STUDENTS WITH OTHER MENTORS?
Physiotherapists		
Podiatrists		
Social workers		
Speech therapists		
Audiologists		
Community health workers		
Radiologists		
Dentists		
Lawyers		
Housing dept.		
Others		

■ *THINK!*

Think about the patient/client's journey from beginning to end. Who will they come into contact with along the way? Make a list and arrange for your student to take the same journey.

■ *THINK!*

You may wish to collect information from other practitioners who have worked with the student to help in their assessment.

Reference / World Health Organization (2010) *Framework for Action on Interprofessional Education and Collaborative Practice*. Geneva: WHO.

■ SUPPORTING STUDENTS WHO HAVE LEARNING DIFFICULTIES

Students who have specific needs will require help and support from their mentors. These students may have specific needs but they will also have individual strengths, which should be acknowledged by the mentor.

Any student who has specific learning difficulties will under the Equality Act (2010) be considered a disabled person. The individual student may not see themselves as disabled. Such a student will be required to achieve the same learning outcomes as other students; however, they may need some adjustments in relation to resources and specific support in order to achieve these. Under the legislation such support is termed reasonable adjustments. Reasonable adjustments will depend upon the needs and difficulties experienced by the individual student. Reasonable adjustments might include modifying working hours, using specific equipment such as a tape recorder, or providing information in an accessible format.

All students are individual regardless of their disability. As a mentor you need to be aware of and understand your responsibilities under the relevant legislation.

As a mentor to a student with learning difficulties you will need to consider the following:

Identification of the student's type of impairment and required support needs – this will be dependent upon the student's level of self-disclosure. Students are usually given the opportunity to disclose a disability on application to a programme.

Discussion with the student of how any disclosed information will be shared with other professionals.

Identification of any equipment the student has already been issued and how this will be utilised in the practice setting.

Identification of how the placement environment can best provide any adjustments required.

Any action plan should include the specific needs and support strategies for the individual student regarding their disability.

A regular review of reasonable adjustments will ensure that they are still providing maximum support.

Equal opportunities are available for all students and there is no discrimination based upon disability.

Facilitate a culture and atmosphere in the workplace which encourages disclosure.

Ensure regular collaboration and discussion with the learner's host educational organisation.

It is useful at the end of the placement for the mentor to seek feedback from the student regarding the support and reasonable adjustments which have been provided.

Reference / Government Equalities Office (2010) *The Equality Act.* London: Equalities Office.

Assessment

The word assessment can have a variety of meanings but an educational assessment refers to the ways in which learning can be measured. You must measure what the student has learnt (knowledge, skills and behaviours) against the standards and learning outcomes which have been set (Minton 1997).

■ THE ASSESSMENT PROCESS

As an assessor, take some time to think through the assessment process and answer the following questions so that you know exactly what it is you are looking for and assessing against.

A FRAMEWORK FOR THE ASSESSMENT PROCESS

What learning outcomes must be achieved to meet the standard required *and* what behaviours should be displayed to be professional?	**Why** is this assessment necessary? Is the student in their first year or at the end of their programme?
How will you assess? Which methods of assessment will demonstrate that the student has achieved the required outcome, question and answer, scenario, observation, reflection, etc.?	**When** is this formative? (The student should be given feedback.) Is it summative? If so, the student should know what is expected of them.

Where will the assessment take place? Is the environment conducive to making a fair assessment? Consider yourself as being part of the environment and remain objective.	**Who** are you assessing? (Know about the student's programme.) Who are *you*, the assessor? Are you up to date as an assessor?

Reference / Minton, D. (1997) *Teaching Skills in Further and Adult Education*, 2nd edn. London: Thomson Learning.

■ INTERVIEWS UNDERTAKEN IN PRACTICE

Interviews require you to establish a personal and professional relationship with your student. A successful interview requires the use of good communication skills.

Pre-meeting preparation

STUDENT'S ROLE
- Students should undertake an appraisal of their own progress and/or competence – against preset outcomes if appropriate.
- Students may use a reflective journal in order to reflect upon their practice.

MENTOR'S ROLE
- Mentors should review the assessment procedures in order to be familiar with the documentation required.
- Mentors should take time to read any evidence presented by the student.

- Mentors should be familiar with the expected level of achievement.
- Mentors should be familiar with the learning outcomes and/or performance criteria to be achieved.

Conduct of interviews
- Interviews should be conducted in private.
- There should be no interruptions.
- Time should be built into the working day to conduct the interview.

INITIAL INTERVIEW
This should take place early in the placement. It may include an orientation to the placement area, if not already undertaken.

This is an opportunity for a discussion between the mentor and the student to establish learning needs, level to be achieved, and set ground rules (see page 8).

Suggested areas for discussion:
- Any special needs identified by the student.
- Learning opportunities within the placement area.
- Opportunities which can be accessed outside the area.
- Times and dates for any subsequent interviews.
- Examination of the required learning outcomes/performance criteria to be achieved.
- An action plan to facilitate achievement of required outcomes.
- Expectations of each other or the placement.

INTERMEDIATE INTERVIEW

This should take place midway through the placement, or earlier if any issues or problems arise. Students can self-assess their knowledge, skills and attitudes in preparation for the interview. Students may be required to undertake self-grading against a set of predefined criteria.

The intermediate interview provides an opportunity to:

- Discuss the student's progress.
- Discuss achievement towards the learning outcomes.
- Discuss any concerns that either the student or mentor has identified.
- Discuss any further learning opportunities required.
- Give and receive feedback.
- Undertake a formative assessment of the student's competence and skills.
- Invite a third person to facilitate the assessment process and clarify issues.
- Set an action plan for the remainder of the placement time.
- Complete any required documentation.

FINAL INTERVIEW

This interview must be completed before the end of the placement period, and will constitute the formal or summative assessment related to the achievement of any specified learning outcomes.

- Students can self-assess their knowledge, skills and attitudes.
- Students may be required to undertake self-grading against a set of predefined criteria.

The final interview provides the opportunity to:
- Discuss the achievement of the learning outcomes.
- Verify that the evidence presented by the student meets the required level/standard.
- Record the mentor's decision as to the achievement of the learning outcomes.
- Identify clearly any learning outcomes not achieved.
- Complete an action plan for the student's continued development – this should be based upon specific and concrete evidence and behaviours.

■ SUPPORTING THE STUDENT WHO IS UNDERACHIEVING

Mentors have recognised the challenge that supporting a student who is underachieving can present. Research undertaken by Duffy (2003) supports this and goes on to identify reasons why mentors may pass students who should fail. These include:
- Awareness of the seriousness of the consequences for the student if they fail them.
- A feeling of personal failure when a learner fails in practice.
- Awareness of a student having personal problems.
- Stress of awarding a fail.
- Giving the student the benefit of the doubt if the student's performance is borderline.

■ *THINK!*

Do you recognise any of these reasons and feelings?

Reference / Duffy, K. (2003) *Failing Students: a qualitative study of factors that influence the decisions regarding assessment of students' competence in practice.* London: NMC.

The mentor cannot relinquish the responsibility and accountability for assessing the student, but there are some things to consider which will help the mentor support the underachieving learner.

- Make an objective assessment of the student by linking their performance to specific learning outcomes.
- Recognise and arrange support for an underachieving student at the earliest opportunity in the placement period.
- Ask colleagues to work with the student and feedback to you as the mentor.
- Communicate to the student any weaknesses/problems regarding their knowledge base, skills, attitudes or behaviour as soon as they are identified.
- Share your concerns with the educational institute.
- Document clearly and concisely the weaknesses of the student's performance linked to the specified outcomes.
- Set specific, measurable objectives linked to outcomes within a documented action plan.

■ ACTION PLANS

You may need to create some objectives for your students, which are defined as action plans. A single action plan should be created for each objective. When creating an action plan for a learner, these should be SMART.

S = Specific
- Objectives must be specific.

M = Measurable
- The objective must be measurable and change behaviour.

A = Achievable
- The objective set must be reachable.
R = Realistic
- Can the objective be achieved, and do you have the resources?
T = Time
- When does the objective need to be achieved?

Reference / http://www.thepracticeofleadership.net/2006/03/11/setting-smart-objectives/

Example of a SMART action plan
By the end of the placement | the junior student | will be able to describe | the importance of eye contact | in conversation with patients or clients.

By the end of the placement – TIME
the junior student – REALISTIC
will be able to describe – MEASURABLE
the importance of eye contact – SPECIFIC
in conversation with patients or clients – ACHIEVABLE

■ FEEDBACK
Giving feedback is essential to a student's learning.
'The old saying that practice makes perfect is not true. But it is true to say that it is practice the results of which are known which makes perfect' (Bartlett 1947 in Rogers 2007 p. 58).

It seems obvious that if you are repeating or practising something which is incorrect, then it will always be incorrect.

If a student is making mistakes, as a mentor you cannot let that continue. You have to tell the student what they are doing wrong and advise them on how to correct it so that they can learn and develop the correct skill, knowledge or behaviour. The way in which feedback is given is also essential to a student's learning.

■ *THINK!*

Can you recall a teacher or mentor who laughed at your attempts to do something or made some cruel remarks?
Can you recall a teacher or mentor who gave you more constructive feedback?
How did you feel and what were the long-term consequences?

Feedback given badly or cruelly can have long-term consequences for the student in that they may give up or be put off the subject for life. Constructive feedback however can inspire and encourage students, especially if they adapt their behaviour and are successful in achieving the desired outcome.

Giving constructive feedback is a higher-level skill and requires self-regulation. The praise sandwich is often used (Gopee 2010), but consider the following section as this will enable your student to reflect on events or incidents and enhance their understanding.

References / Gopee, N. (2010) *Practice Teaching in Healthcare*. London: Sage; Rogers, J. (2007) *Adults Learning*, 5th edn. Maidenhead: OUP McGraw-Hill Education.

Feedback guidelines
Use the following framework to support you when giving feedback.

QUESTIONS BASED UPON GOOD PRACTICE GUIDANCE	COMMENTS ON THE FEEDBACK GIVEN
Limit your feedback to what was actually observed, e.g. *'I noticed that you did not explain the procedure to the patient.'*	
Feedback should test out what had been heard or seen, e.g. *'It appeared to me that the patient was anxious'*.	
Do not make assumptions about what had been seen or heard: you may be wrong.	
Focus on how the situation made *you* feel rather than judging if the behaviour/ issue was good or bad, e.g. *'I felt embarrassed when you spoke sharply to the patient.'*	
Do not give personal opinions on the issue.	

QUESTIONS BASED UPON GOOD PRACTICE GUIDANCE	COMMENTS ON THE FEEDBACK GIVEN
Limit the number of points identified so that you do not overwhelm the receiver.	
Be specific and focused, e.g. *'When you said . . . ?' 'When you did . . . ?' 'I noticed that . . . ?'*	
Help the receiver reflect on how others see or hear them, e.g. *'How do you think the patient felt?'*	
Use questions to seek information, e.g. *'Can you clarify for me what was happening when you . . . ?'*	
Do not use feedback in such a manner as to criticise or manipulate the receiver.	
Consider if the feedback is likely to alter the receiver's behaviour.	
Consider if the feedback was helpful for the receiver.	

References / Adapted from Aldridge, S. and Rigby, S. (2000) *Counselling Skills in Context.* London: Hodder & Stoughton.

■ COMPLETING DOCUMENTATION (RECORDS OF PROGRESS)

Record keeping should follow any organisational/ professional requirements and guidelines. Where a signature is required the person's usual full signature should be used.

Completed documentation regarding a student's progress should:

- Contain evidence of student's orientation to the placement area.
- Contain evidence of any formal interviews undertaken.
- Contain evidence of clear and concise action planning.
- If applicable, record the verification of hours undertaken by the student.
- Identify evidence supporting claims for achievement of learning outcomes/performance criteria.
- Record the mentor's verification that the student has or has not achieved the relevant learning outcomes.

■ JUSTIFYING ASSESSMENT DECISIONS

In order to justify an assessment decision it is important to have a systematic approach to the process so that you can identify exactly what has been good about the student's performance and what has not. As a guide in your decision making, a checklist and a progressive assessment framework will be helpful.

A checklist can help you isolate the component parts of the performance.

■ *THINK!*

Consider the following:

NAME:	YES / NO	COMMENTS
Standard of practice Has the student demonstrated safe and effective practice throughout?		
Application of theory to practice Do you have evidence that the student integrates theory and practice?		
Level of knowledge Does the student have sound knowledge and understanding of practice?		
Critical analysis Does the student use evidence to critically analyse situations which occur in practice and service provision?		
Receiving and responding Does the student actively seek out opportunities to develop their learning and demonstrate independent thinking?		
Value complex Are they enthusiastic, motivated, eager to contribute to developing practice?		

Reference / Adapted from Bloom, B.S. (ed.) (1956) *Taxonomy of Educational Objectives, the classification of educational goals – Handbook I: Cognitive Domain.* New York: McKay.

A progressive assessment framework appears in *The Experiential Taxonomy* (Steinaker and Bell 1979). The principles of the framework can also be used to determine the level expected of the student and provide the focus for assessing practice. Identification and internalisation are described separately but often happen together.

NAME:	COMMENTS
Exposure What were your observations of the student? How did the student react to the experience? Did they have an understanding of events and terminology and were they able to describe what was happening? Were they keen to engage?	
Participation Were they able to describe how they would do it if given the opportunity? Was the student able to assist in the activity or the experience?	
Identification and internalisation Can the student carry out the activity under supervision and demonstrate an understanding of the rationale behind it? Have you used different methods to assess their understanding?	

NAME:	COMMENTS
Dissemination Is the student able to transfer their skills and knowledge to different situations? Do they work as part of the team and organise their work accordingly? Are they beginning to act as a role model and teach others?	
Extend your assessment and consider others' views	
Feedback What feedback has the student had from other members of the team, managers and patients/clients? Has the feedback you have given to the student been applied?	

Reference / Adapted from Steinaker, N. and Bell, M. (1979) *The Experiential Taxonomy: a new approach to teaching and learning.* New York: Academic Press.

Accountability and responsibility

As a qualified practitioner you are **accountable** to:

Profession – your professional body.

Employer – you have signed a contract with them and must abide by their policies and procedures.

The law of the land – any action you take which is illegal will be dealt with accordingly.

In addition, a mentor may also feel **responsible** to:

Profession – you want to contribute to the development of a future workforce which will not only maintain high professional standards but also add value to the profession, and you want to be able to contribute to the workforce as a trusted colleague.

Student – you want your student to achieve their potential and be the best that they can be.

Yourself – being a mentor is a very rewarding role. It can enhance and inspire you but can also be demanding and challenging, especially when a student is not achieving their learning outcomes.

Mentors are very aware of their accountability and responsibility, and work by Orland-Barak (2002) identified that mentors often felt that they were pulled in different directions. They recognised that they had multiple roles – the mentor as a person, as a professional and as a teacher and assessor. Occasionally tension arises when there appears to be conflict between these roles, which can cause anxiety for the mentor and the student.

> ***Concern** – mentors can feel that they are to blame if a student fails.

Remember, mentors cannot force their students to learn: they can only facilitate their learning (Rogers 1969). Therefore if you have created an appropriate learning environment for your student and have provided them with the resources they need to learn, you have acted responsibly.

*Concern – mentors may feel that if they pass their student at the point of registration, and the student later goes on to commit illegal or unprofessional acts, they may themselves be called to account and disciplined.

Remember, once qualified, your former student is accountable and responsible for their behaviour.

■ *THINK!*

Consider this. If you were driving home tonight and had an accident in your car, would you sue the driving instructor with whom you had passed your test?

If a formal investigation was held regarding a former student you might be asked if you noticed any behaviours or attitudes that were unusual (which reinforces the reasons why it is important to keep clear records) but you would not be held responsible for the choices or actions another qualified individual makes.

References / Orland-Barak, L. (2002) What's in a case: what mentors' cases reveal about the practice of mentoring. *Journal of Curriculum Studies* 34(4), 451–68; Rogers, C.R. (1969) *Freedom to Learn*. Columbus, OH: Charles E. Merrill Publishing Co.

Evaluation

Evaluation is a part of the quality assurance process. It is the process of obtaining information which identifies strengths and weaknesses associated with:

- **The teaching and learning process**
  This evaluation can include performance of mentors and other practitioners, as well as of physical and practical resources.

- **The learning environment**
  Asking students to evaluate the strengths and weaknesses of the placement environment, as a source of learning opportunities.

- **The mentor**
  The mentor may invite the student to offer evaluative feedback on their performance as a mentor.

  Mentors can also undertake a self-evaluation of their performance. This enables the mentor to continue to improve their role.

- **The assessment process and documentation**
  The mentor and student can evaluate the usefulness and validity of the assessment process and associated documentation.

  Students may undertake a formal evaluation of their practice experience when returning to their education institution. It is also valuable for mentors in placement areas to design a student evaluation tool to collect their own information for evaluation.

Updating and ongoing development

It is acknowledged (NMC 2008) that in order to provide quality mentorship, professionals who undertake this role need to engage in life-long learning and updating. The NMC (2008) have a mandatory requirement for updating, and the following advice is based upon those standards.

The following are identified areas which relate to the updating:

Knowledge – the need to keep up to date in respect of

a) Requirements for mentor competence as described by own professional body.

b) Changes and amendments to learners' training programmes, especially those that impact on practice and mentor role.

Competence – the need to practise mentorship skills by supporting and assessing students regularly.

NMC (2008) require mentors to have evidence of acting in a mentor role for a minimum of two students in a three-year period.

Competence can also be developed by discussing the experiences of assessing in practice as a group activity.

Self-assessment – the need to examine own performance and accountability.

To plan ongoing mentor development, in order to meet professional standards for learning and assessing in practice.

Peer assessment – independent professional review of mentor skills and competence.

Explore mentorship role as a group activity.

Meet with line manager to review performance. NMC (2008) require this to occur at least once every three years.

Maintain professional requirements – the need to meet specified professional requirements. To be registered on a local database of mentors if this exists.

Meet requirements specified by service providers in order to remain on the database.

All of the above could be achieved by:

a) Attendance at updating workshops.

b) Completing a recognised workbook, hard copy or on-line.

c) Spending time with other mentors discussing the role and the assessment process.

d) Recording your evidence of mentor activities such as type of updates attended, number of students mentored.

e) Peer review of assessment documentation.

References / Nursing & Midwifery Council (2008) *Standards to support learning and assessment in practice: NMC standards for mentors, practice teachers and teachers*, 2nd edn. London: NMC.

■ CASE STUDIES THAT COULD BE DISCUSSED WITH A GROUP OF MENTORS

Case (a)

A student regularly arrives late for practice and gives a range of reasons for this lateness. The student has been made aware of the importance of arriving on time but still persists in arriving late.

As a mentor how would you deal with this situation?

You may want to refer to the following: feedback guidelines; ground rules; action planning; completing documentation; accountability.

Case (b)
Your student is enthusiastic and motivated; however, they are having difficulty in achieving some of the required learning outcomes for their placement.
Explore what would be the strategies you could use to support the student.
You may want to refer to the following: learning styles; learning theories; supporting an underachieving student; supporting a student with learning difficulties.

Case (c)
You are a mentor supporting a final-year student. The student identifies at the initial interview that she needs to develop her management skills.
i) Plan how you are going to address this.
ii) Discuss how you will assess her progress.
You may want to refer to the following: the assessment process; justifying assessment decisions; the interview process; action planning; inter-professional learning; evaluation.

■ SELF-EVALUATION

Darling (1985) identified styles of mentoring which could have a negative effect upon the student and could be detrimental to the student's learning.

■ *THINK!*

Read through the following negative styles and make sure that you are developing a style which facilitates a positive learning experience for students in placement.

- **Avoiders/ignorers/non-responders** – mentors who are hard to contact, often unavailable or inaccessible.
- **Dumpers** – mentors who 'throw people into the deep end', exposing them to new situations without support, a 'sink or swim' approach.
- **Blockers** – control by withholding information or refusing requests. Development can be suppressed by over-supervising.
- **Destroyers/criticisers** – subtle attacks which erode confidence and humiliate the student. Public verbal criticism questioning ability and destroying confidence.

Reference / Darling, L.A. (1985) What to do about toxic mentors. *Journal of Nursing Administration* **15**(5), 43–4.

■ *THINK!*

As a mentor, consider self-evaluation:

What are your strengths? Name two	a)	b)
What are your weaknesses? Name two	a)	b)
What could occur that may prevent you from being a good mentor?	a)	b)
How could you overcome these barriers?	a)	b)

■ REFLECTION

Reflection can be a useful tool on many levels:

a) To help the mentor become more self-aware by examining their role and performance.

b) As a teaching and learning process.

a) Self-awareness

Reflection can give you the time to think through your feelings and actions as a mentor.

You can do this by sharing and reflecting with other mentors or by keeping a written journal. In this you can describe a significant event or experience and then examine this to see why you acted in a certain way and if you could do things differently another time.

b) Teaching tool

Reflection can be utilised with students to help them develop their performance and professionalism.

If you take time with your student to debrief after an event it will allow them to gather their thoughts and feelings. Looking back on the experience can allow them with guidance to consider their or others' actions. By considering the event in depth it can increase their understanding and awareness.

■ *THINK!*

How would you do this with your student?

DISCUSSION

1. Choose an event or experience.
2. Ask the student to think about it.
3. Then with the student go through the event in detail, reviewing the actions and why they occurred.
4. Explore alternative actions that could have been taken.
5. Identify new insights that could be utilised in a similar event.

WRITTEN JOURNAL/DIARY

You could also ask your student to write a reflective journal/diary. This is a record accurately describing an event and then evaluating the event, exploring new actions which could be taken.

The student could be encouraged to think about the following questions when reflecting by either process.

- What did I do?
- Why did I take that action?
- What evidence supported my action?
- How successful was the action?
- What else could I have done?
- What would I do next time?

There are a range of theoretical models which you could utilise to lead your reflection. Some of these are identified below:

- **Kolb's learning cycle** (Kolb, D.A. (1984) *Experiential learning; experience as the source of learning*. New Jersey: Prentice-Hall).
- **Gibb's reflective cycle** (Gibbs, G. (1988) *Learning by doing: a guide to teaching and learning methods*. Oxford: Oxford Brookes University).

- **Atkins and Murphy's model of reflection** (Atkins, S., Murphy, K. (1994) Reflective Practice. *Nursing Standard* **8**(39), 49–56).
- **John's model of structured reflection** (John, C., Graham, J. (1996) Using a reflective model of nursing and guided reflection. *Nursing Standard* **11**(2), 34–8).

Summary of learning theories

LEARNING THEORY	DESIRED OUTCOME	EXAMPLE	STRATEGY
Behaviourist approach	Useful for (psychomotor) activity which requires the student to act quickly and where knowledge (cognitive) is required instantly	Giving injections Basic life support Making a diagnosis	Demonstration and regular practice Rote learning Mnemonics Acronyms Chants or rhymes
Social learning theory	Developing skills and qualities Psychomotor and affective domain	Communication Professional behaviour	Role modelling Talking through a procedure to promote self-regulation

Summary of learning theories (*continued*)

LEARNING THEORY	DESIRED OUTCOME	EXAMPLE	STRATEGY
Cognitive	Knowledge and understanding Self-regulation Self-monitoring	Applying theory to practice Critical analysis Workload planning Change management Problem-solving	Determining the student's preferred learning style Facilitating experiences that enable the student to explore the issues or the process, e.g. break the process down into its component parts and build them up again Writing a portfolio
Humanist	Lifelong learner Self awareness	Comprehending concepts Collaborative working Autonomy	Reflection Debate Experiential learning Scenarios/case studies

Glossary

Assessment: a measure by which achievement is compared to a pre-set standard.

Capability: not just what you do in your current situation but also how you can transfer your ability to different situations.

Competence: the ability to perform a specific task, action or function successfully.

Evaluation: a systematic process that is designed to provide information that will help develop and improve a situation.

Inter-professional learning: the process of practitioners from a range of professions learning from each other's roles.

Lifelong learning: continued professional and personal development.

Learning outcome: the required standard of achievement.

Learning styles: the individual's preferred approach to learning.

Mentor: a qualified practitioner responsible for teaching and assessing students.

Placement: a workplace learning environment.

Practitioner: qualified professional member of staff.

Self-awareness: understanding the impact your behaviour has on others.

Self-regulated learning: the ability to reflect in and on actions and to monitor your own performance.

Student: an individual undertaking a programme/module of study.

Record of annual update

Evidence of updating

DATE	TYPE OF ACTIVITY

See section Updating and ongoing development on pp. 38–44.

Record of individual students

NAME AND DATE	LEVEL

Other things to remember

Important phone numbers and email addresses

NAME	PHONE NO.	EMAIL